Easy Exercises Sitting in a Chair –for the Elderly, Office Workers and Others Who have Neglected Their Fitness

By Ken Ward

Copyright

Copyright © 2019 Kenneth J Ward, Leigh-on-Sea, United Kingdom (Author and Artist)
All Rights Reserved
This book is an original work (text and images.)

Contents

Easy Exercises Sitting in a Chair –for the Elderly, Office Workers and Others Who have Neglected Their Fitness 1
By Ken Ward 1
   Copyright 2
   Contents 3
   Important 6
You need… 6
   Advantages of Chair Exercises 7
   Origin of the Exercises. 8
   How to Use This Book 10
A Journey Through the Body 11
   THE EXERCISES 12
   Base Position 13
   Ankles and Feet 15
Toes Up 15
Heels Up 16
Feet Turned Outwards 17
Feet Turned Inward 18
   Legs and Thighs 19
Knee Up 19
Legs Spread 21
Legs Spread Against Resistance 22
Legs Closing Against Resistance 23
One Leg Crossed while Bending Forward 24
Cross Your Legs and Raise Your Lower Leg 25

Leg Straight Out 27
Leg Straight Out Supported 28
Figure Four Exercise 29
   Back 31
Bend Back 31
Bend Forward 32
   Side Bends 34
Start Position 34
Bend Right and Left 35
    Bend Right 35
    Bend Left 36
   Body Twists 37
Twist Right 37
   Alternative Body Twists 39
Fingers on Shoulders (Base Position) 39
Twist Right 41
Twist Left 42
    Belly Muscles (Abs) 43
    Arms and Shoulders 45
Hands Behind Head 45
Arms Up 47
Arms T pose 48
Arms Straight Out 49
Reversed Arms Stretch 50
Shrugs 51
Elbow Circles 52
   Hands 53
Hands Spread 54

Hands Fists 55
  Prayer Hand Poses 56
Prayer Hands Middle 57
Prayer Hands Down 57
Prayer Hands Up 58
Prayer Hands Right 58
Prayer Hands Left 59

  Neck 60
Finger-tip Pressure 60
Head Bent Back 61
Head Bent Forward 61
Look Left 62
Look Right 63

  Eyes 65
Eyes Straight Ahead 65
Eyes Right 66
Eyes Up 66
Eyes Left 67
Eyes Down 67

  Heart and Lungs (Aerobic Exercises.) 68
Raising Your Knees 68
Raising Your Knees and Arms 70

  The Future 72

Important

Consult your health-care provider before embarking on an exercise plan.
- Do the exercises *slowly* and *gently*.
- Exit poses gradually. Relax your muscles and flow into the relaxed position.
- Hold all extremes in a comfortable position: never with pain and never force them. Avoid exercises that do not suit you.
- Keep Breathing! It is easy to concentrate on the exercise and hold your breath. Try to breathe normally.

You need…
- A safe, stable chair.
- If you are fragile, you should have another person present, should you need help
- Wear suitable clothes and shoes. Wear shoes and loose clothing. (The models in this book do not always do this in order to show the poses more clearly.) This is optional really, but it's common sense.

Advantages of Chair Exercises

- The exercises can be begun comfortably and at your own pace.
- It seems **safer** to do exercises in a chair, especially if you have balance problems.
- Some say **you are less likely to have accidents and injuries** if you strengthen your muscles before embarking on, say, jogging and other exercises.
- **If you are frail**, exercising in a chair may be your only resort, if your health-care provider agrees.
- **If you are fit, but pressed for time**, chair exercises might be for you.
- This book does **not** require you to have any **equipment** except a chair, or even the side of your bed.

Going to a gym and having a personal trainer may be better, but at first you might value:
- Avoiding time and trouble travelling to the gym.
- You may have nobody watching you.
- You save money on fees and travel.

8

Origin of the Exercises.

Thousands of years ago, various exercise systems were developed throughout the world; for instance, *yoga*, *qigong* and *tai chi chuan*.

In yoga, etc, the stances were composed of other exercises combined to form the full poses. This enabled the yogi to do exercises for several muscles at the same time or in the same set.

The following example illustration is taken from 'The Little Book of Qigong" by Ken Ward (the author of this book.) It shows how several parts of the body are exercised in one set.

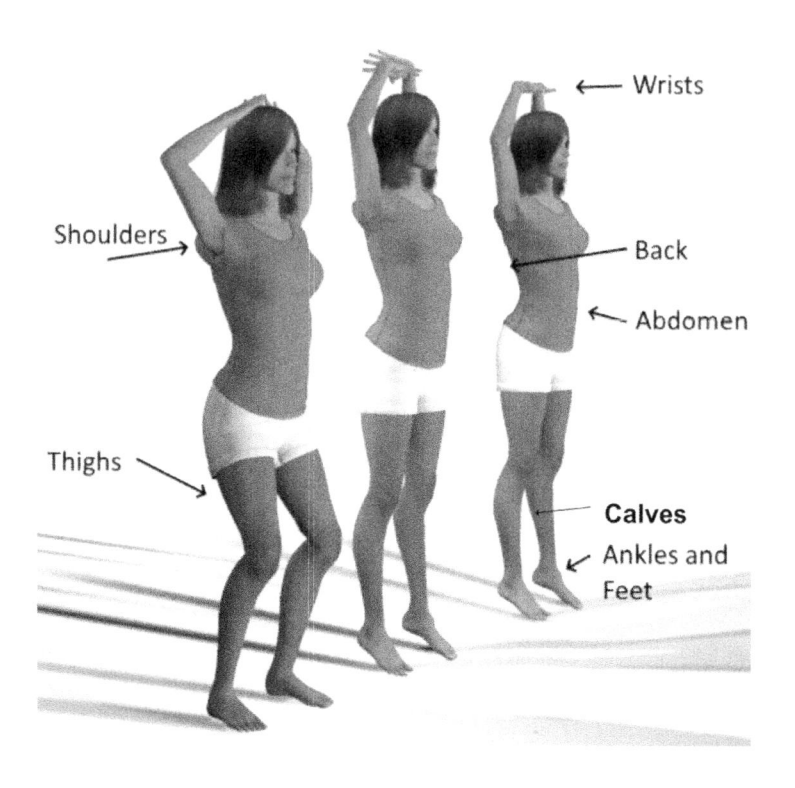

9

(You won't be asked to do such poses in this book!)

While qigong, tai chi chuan and yoga are excellent they may be too difficult, at first, for a beginner. Hence in this book the poses are (usually) exercises for one part of the body so they are simple and easy to learn. They are all done sitting in a chair.

For instance, the exercises for the ankles are done in separate exercises, sitting in a chair.

The toes up and heels up are two of the exercises dealing mainly with the ankles.

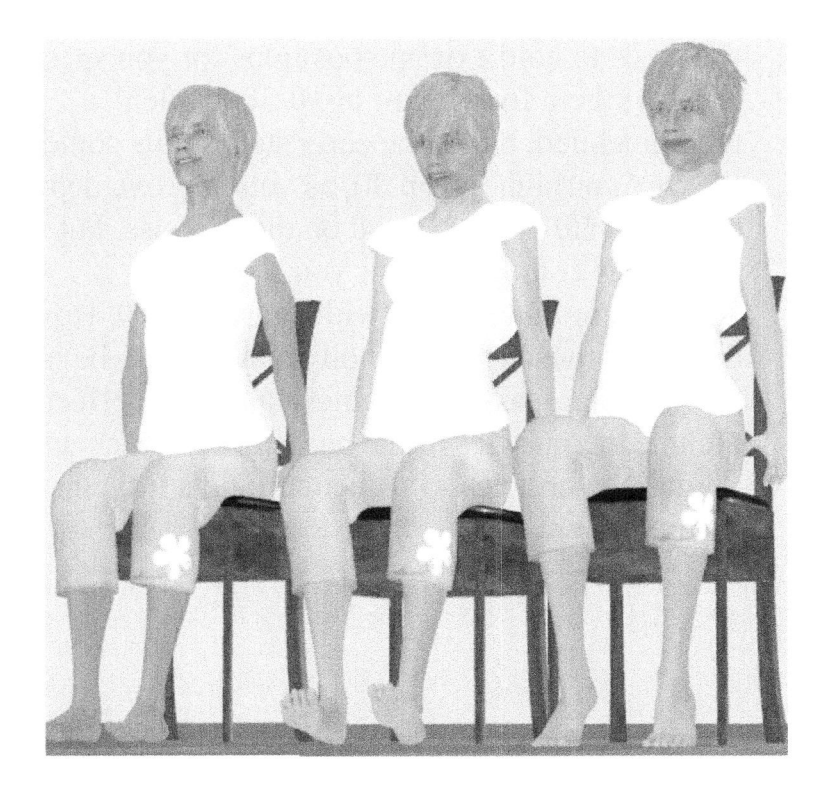

How to Use This Book

You need to learn the exercises by practising them gently and slowly. When you have learned the exercises, it will take about ten to twenty minutes to do them.

Because everyone is different, except by chance, the illustrations are not of a person with your proportions and state of flexibility: different folk have different body proportions and flexibility.

When first reading and learning the exercises, you learn the times to hold extreme positions for you specifically. Holding them for a count of 10-30 is often recommended, but in the early stages, this could be as low as 5, or higher than 30, as you improve depending on your state of fitness and on the exercise, but mostly on what is comfortable for you.

As a rule of thumb, start with a count of 10. However, the larger muscles of the body may need to be held for a count of at least 30 to achieve a training effect. These include the muscles of the backside, stomach and thighs. Nevertheless, it is better to do a little than to do nothing.

A Journey Through the Body

Consider the learning period as a journey through your body. Mentally, look inside and feel the effects of the exercises as you learn them. This is mindfulness and it is how the ancients learned these exercises.

THE EXERCISES

Base Position

Sit straight in the chair and relax:
- Breathing naturally
- Arms by your sides
- Knees vertically in line with your feet
- Your belly-button pulled in (where possible).

Hold the position below for a count of 30 (or longer.)

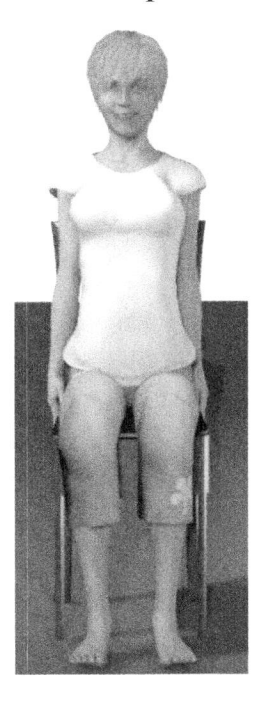

How did you feel? Did your shoulders feel relaxed (even though there may be some muscle tension as they learn the relaxed position?)
How did your belly feel holding your abdominal muscles in?

As always, you can adjust this position to suit your current state of fitness.

Ankles and Feet

Do these slowly, always comfortably. Think into your body and make adjustments as necessary to your poses.

Toes Up

Sitting in the base position (holding onto the chair if necessary) raise your toes from the floor by bending your ankles. Hold for a count of 10-30.

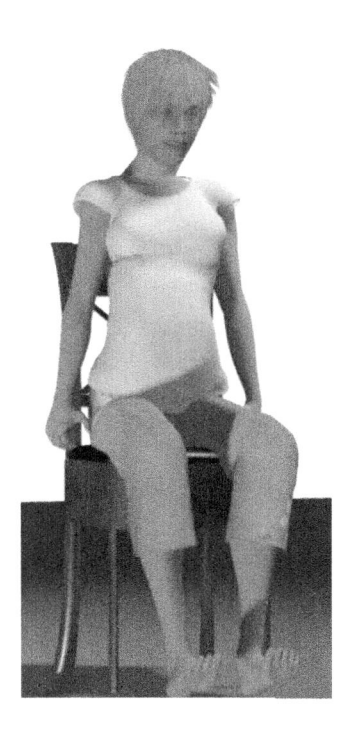

Did you notice the effect on your lower legs, including your calves and toes? (Slow and comfortable–as always.)

Heels Up

Similar to Toes Up. Raise your heels and keep your toes in contact with the floor.

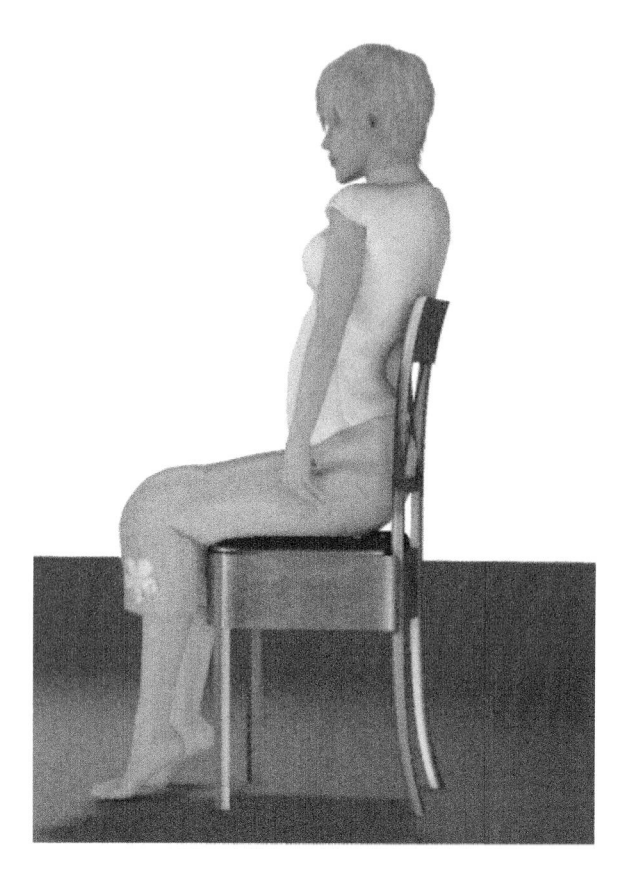

Toes, lower legs, thighs and bum muscles may feel this.

Feet Turned Outwards

Start with your feet flat on the floor. Keep them vertically below your knees and turn your feet outwards. Hold this stretch for a count of 10 to 30.

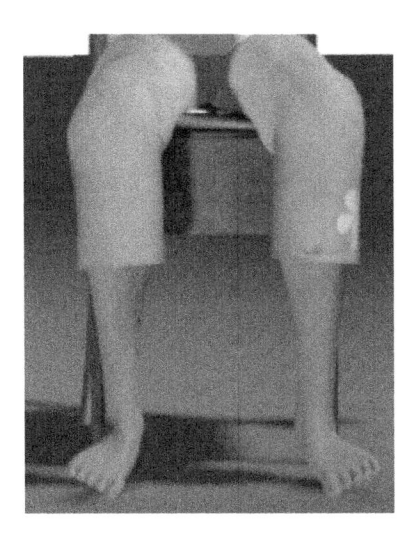

You should feel the stretch in your ankles, in this and the following pose.

Feet Turned Inward

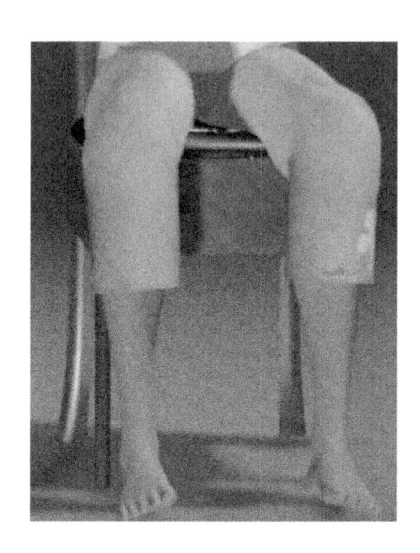

Legs and Thighs

Knee Up
Raise your right knee, holding onto the chair if necessary. Hold for a count of 10-30.

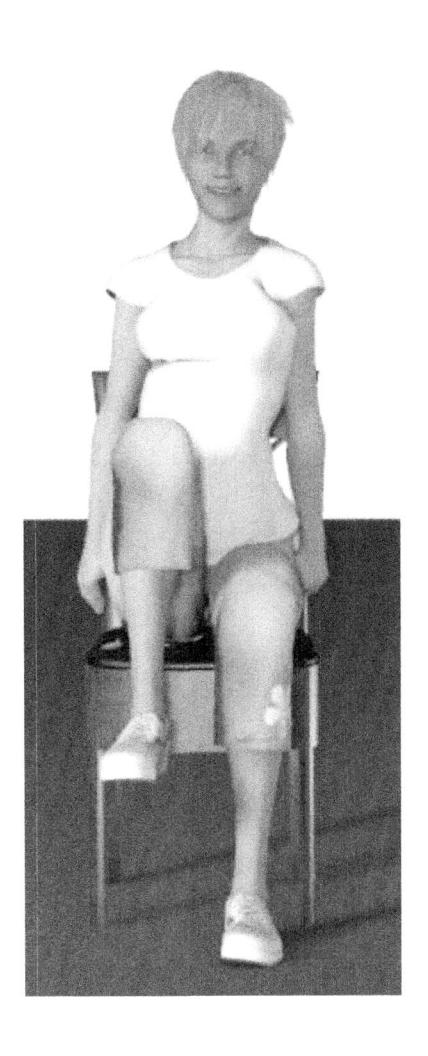

Repeat for your left leg.

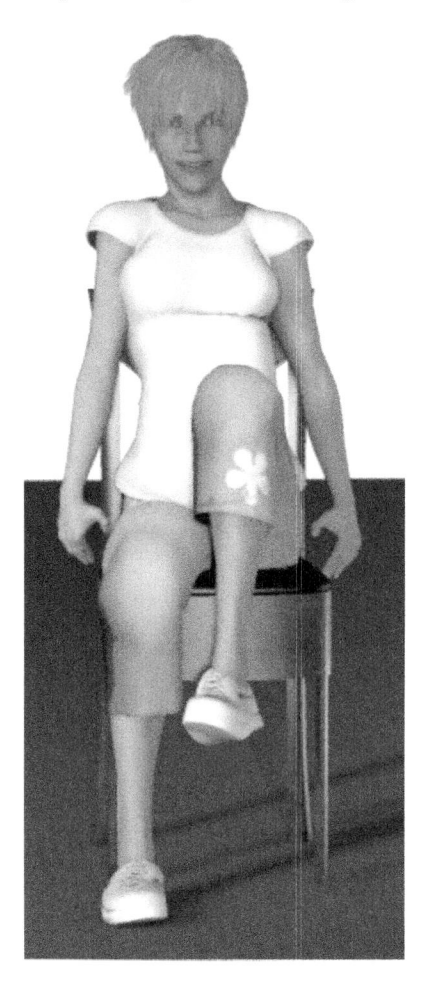

These poses affect your thighs. Although you may also notice tension in your feet, it is possible to mentally relax your feet and concentrate on your thighs, but this is an option. If not, your feet get exercised too.

Legs Spread

Keep your feet flat on the floor and in line with your knees, and your spine straight. Spread your legs (man-spread) as far as is comfortable. If you can, gently press your legs further apart with your hands. The closer to your knee you press, the more the pressure.

It may be possible to wriggle your legs out further as your muscles and tendons relax. Hold for a count of 10-30. These muscles respond better to a longer count. If it is comfortable to do so, hold the pose longer.

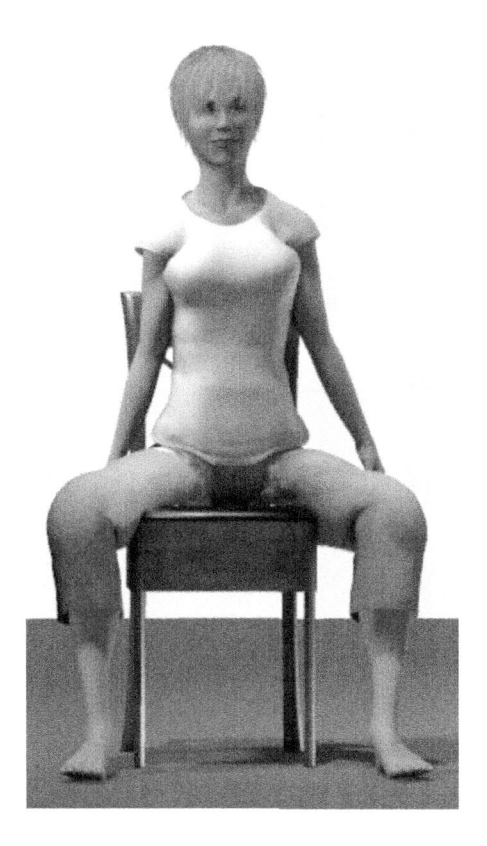

The stretch is felt in your inner thighs. If you can hold this position for, say, a count of 20-30, you may find your legs can be spread out further during the exercise.

Legs Spread Against Resistance

Slowly spread your legs to a comfortable position then apply resistance with your hands. Hold for a count of 10-30.

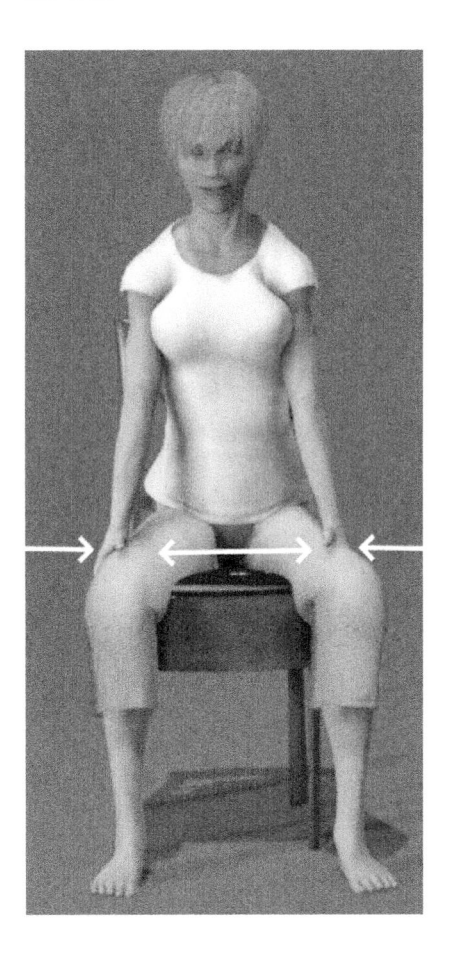

Legs Closing Against Resistance

Keep your feet flat on the floor and in line with your knees, and your spine straight. Try to close your legs while resisting the force with your hands. The closer to your knee you press, the more the pressure.
Hold for a count of 10-30.

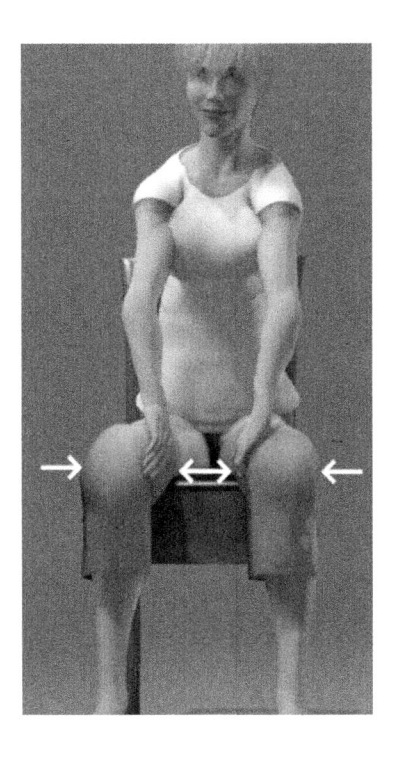

You may feel these exercises affecting your upper thigh muscles between your legs.

One Leg Crossed while Bending Forward

Cross your right leg over your left leg. Move your left foot to your right, as is comfortable for you.
Bend forwards.
Hold for a count of 10 to 50, holding for 30 if possible.
Repeat for your left leg.

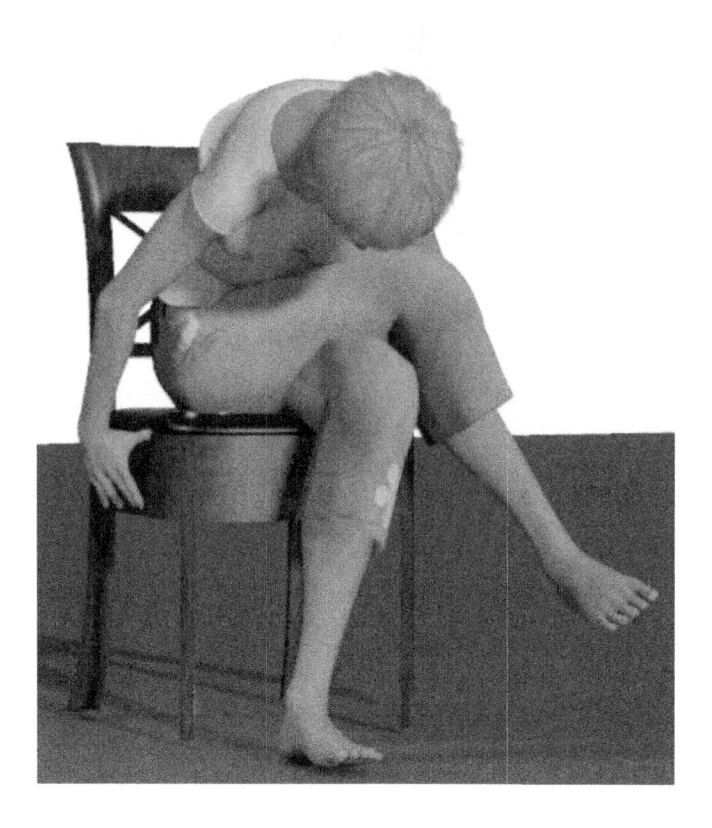

This affects your right upper thigh muscles and bum (glutes). Crossing your left leg and bending it affects the corresponding muscles on your left

Cross Your Legs and Raise Your Lower Leg

Begin by crossing your right leg:

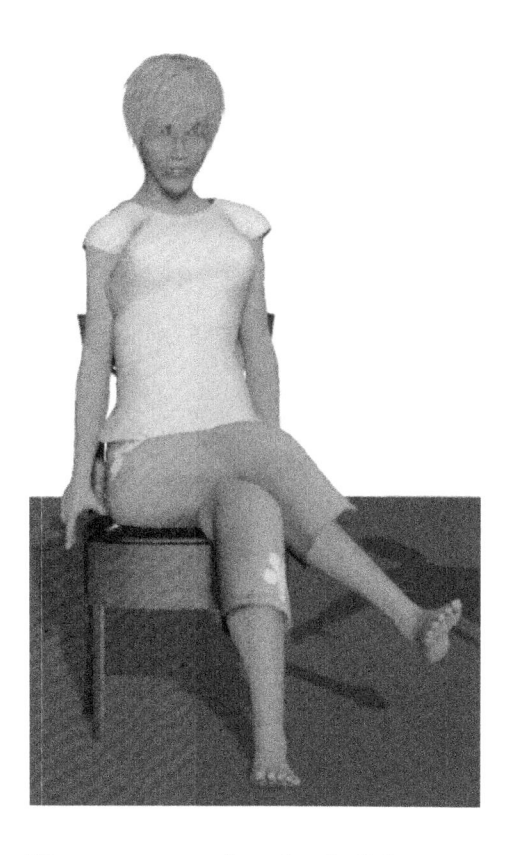

Then try to raise the left leg.

Raise your left leg.

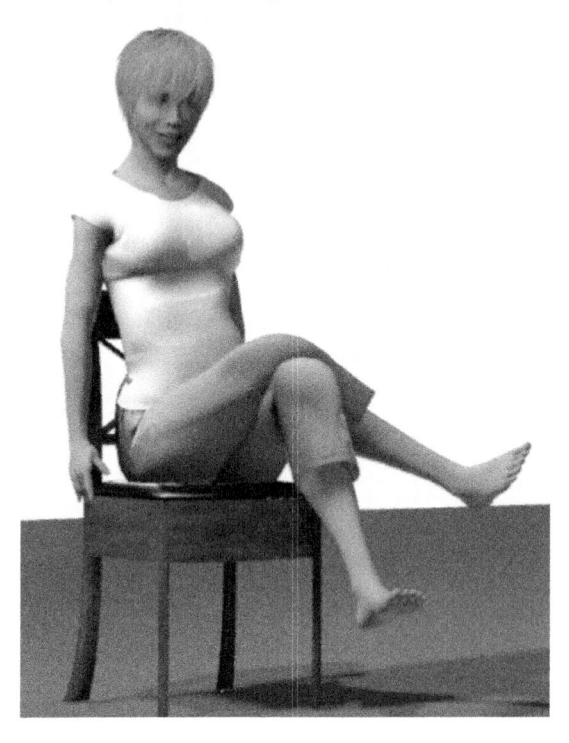

If you find you can raise your left leg only a little, then that is fine.
There may be almost no movement when trying to raise your left leg– you just feel your stretch. At first, do the best you comfortably can.
Hold this pose for a count of 5 to 30.
You may notice the stretch in the side of your bum and the upper thigh of your left leg.
Repeat for your right leg.

Leg Straight Out

You simply stick your right leg out straight. Hold for a count of 10-30. Repeat for your left leg.

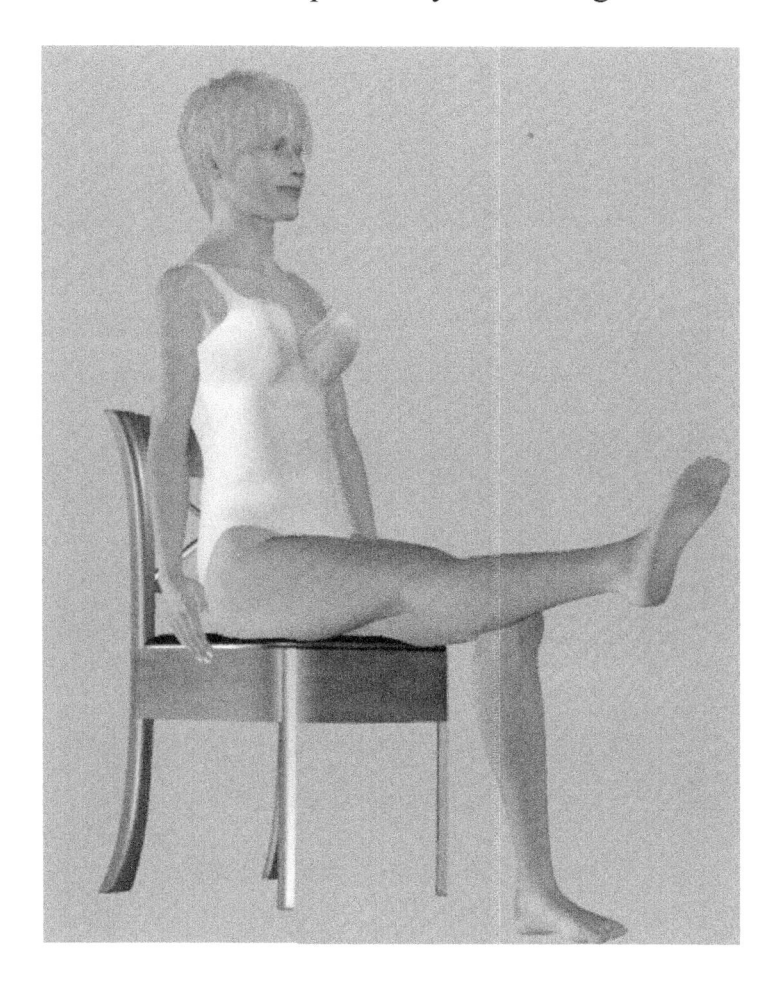

This is felt mainly in your thighs. Repeat for your other leg.

Leg Straight Out Supported
At first you can support your extended leg lightly to support your leg.

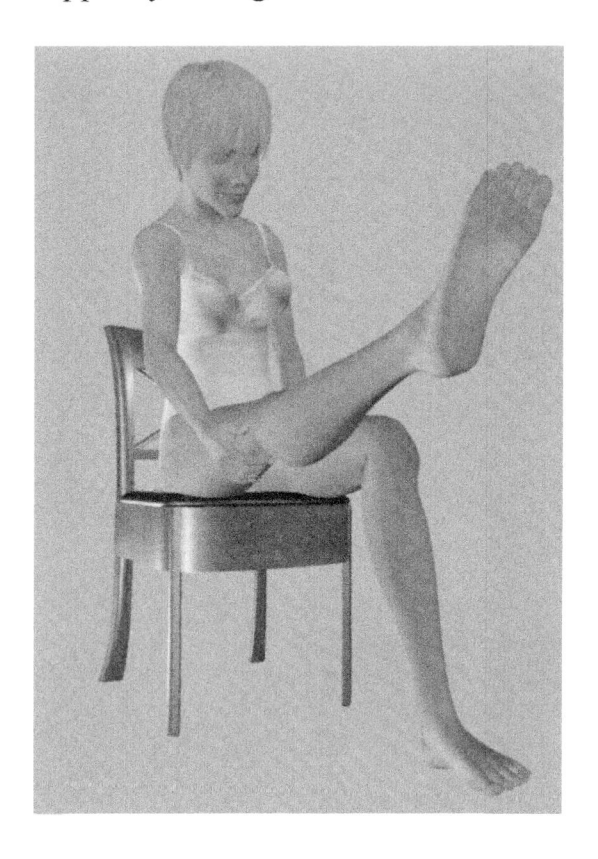

Figure Four Exercise

Put one leg over your other, as when sitting cross legged. Sit a bit forward in the chair so nothing is supporting your lower leg. Press gently on your lower thigh or knee. Hold for a count of 30 if you can. Your leg may bend further during the exercise and as other muscles relax. Repeat for the other leg.

Right Leg

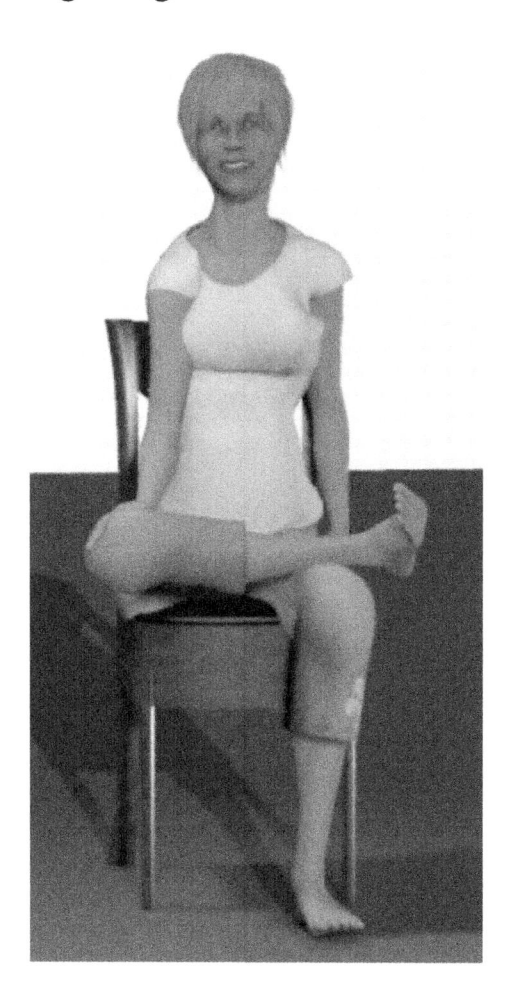

30

Left Leg

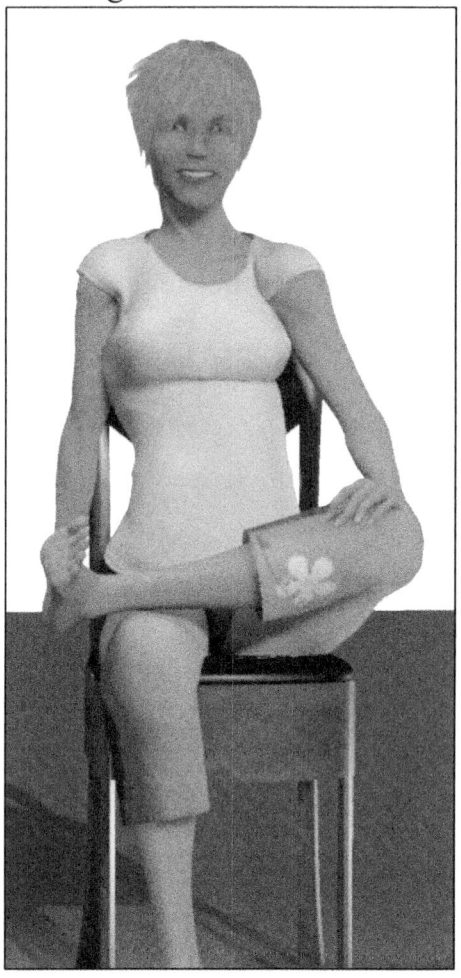

One leg is often more flexible than your other at first so don't be surprised if one leg bends more than the other.

This exercise affects your upper thighs and hip muscles of your bent leg.

Back

Bend Back

Sit a bit forward in the chair and raise your arms and lean back. This is a natural movement to reduce tension (as well as stretching your arms and back.) Hold for a count of 1-30.
(Don't use the back of the chair to support you: it could topple.)
Repeat 3 to 5 times.

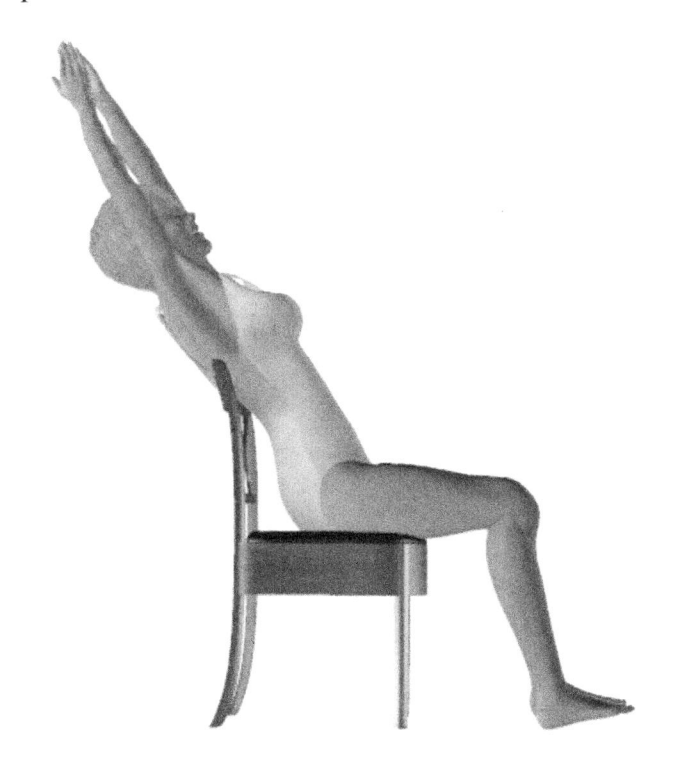

Notice the effects on your arms, back and sides. Notice for yourself how it affects other parts of your body.

Bend Forward

Lean forward, reaching for your feet. How far you can stretch depends on your anatomy. You should stretch just as far as is comfortable. Some people can reach as far as in the floor. Others can reach only to their shins. Do what you comfortably can at first. Try to hold the extreme position for a count of 30.

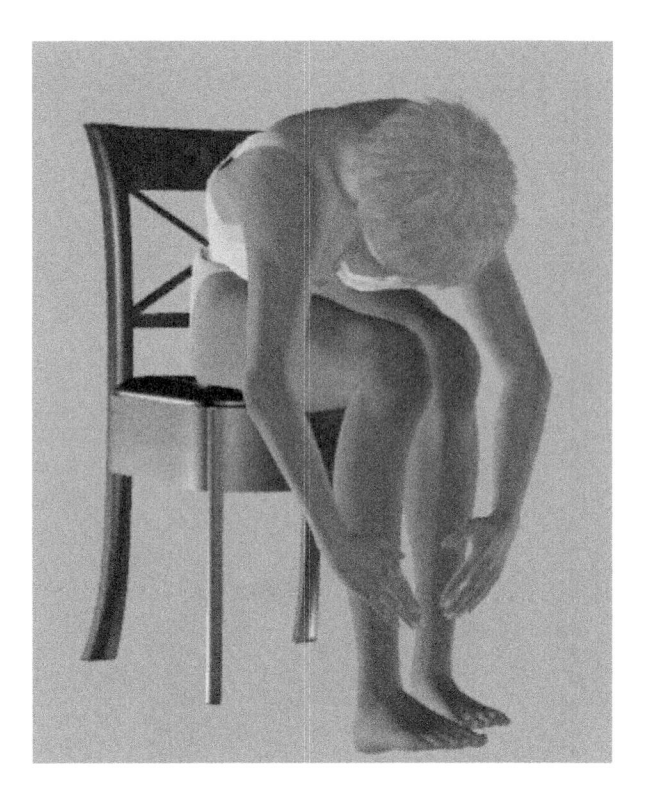

Your back is stimulated when you bend. As your spine isn't under load, most healthy people can bend their spine safely (We do it all the time.)

If your health advisor agrees, you could try this exercise if you feel dizzy when bending from a standing position.

Side Bends

Remember, "*slowly, comfortably* and *without pain.*"

Start Position

Sit with your feet thigh-width apart and knees vertically above your feet. Keep your spine straight.
Stretch your arms above your head or as far as it is comfortable.
Hold for a count of 10-30.

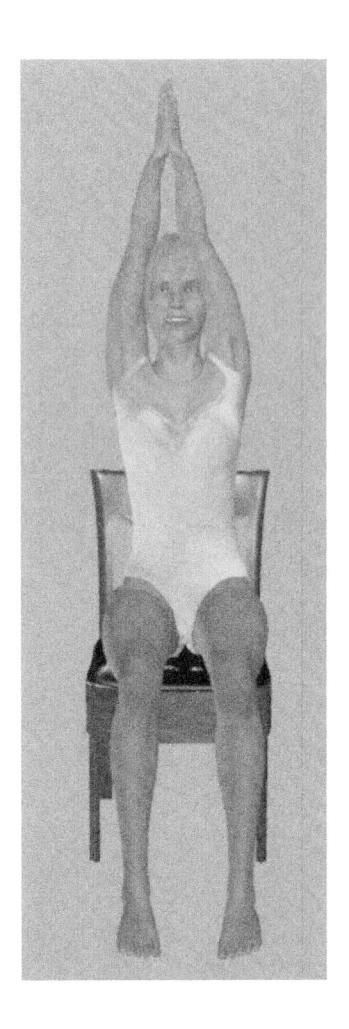

Bend Right and Left

Bend to your right, bending your waist and chest mainly. Hold for a count of 10-30. Repeat for your left side.

Bend Right

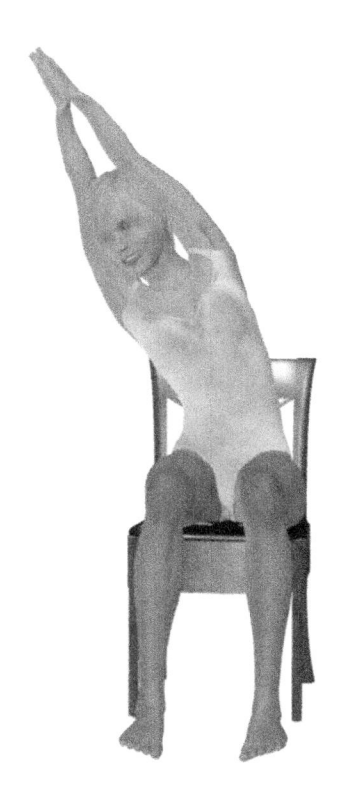

You may mainly feel the stretch on your left side. Scan your body to notice if other muscles are awakened.

Bend Left

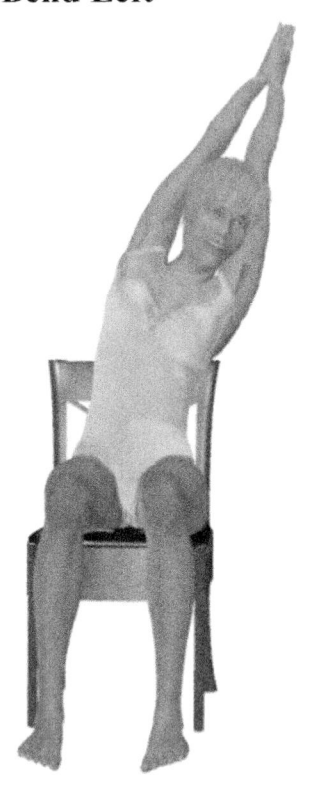

You may feel the stretch mainly on the right side.

Body Twists

See also: Alternative Body Twists.

Twist Right

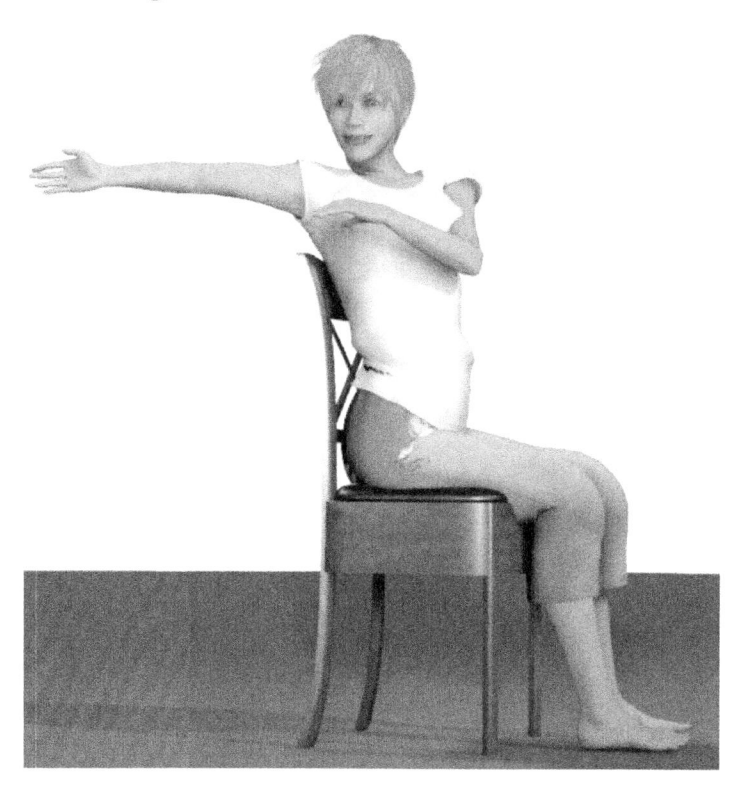

Twist your head and shoulders to your right keeping your spine straight and twisting your waist, chest, neck and head. Hold for a count of 10-30. Repeat for your right side.
Twist Right

Twist Left

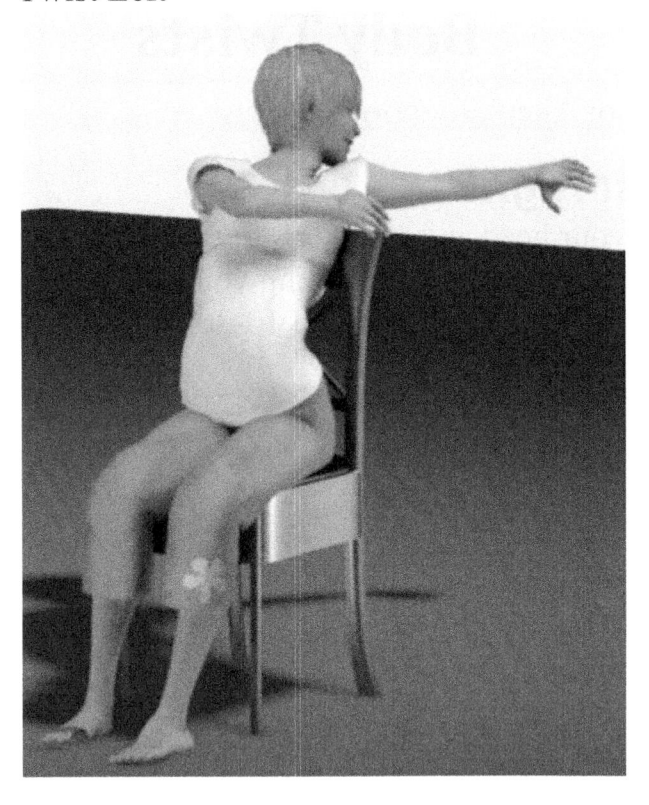

Alternative Body Twists

I added these because the other twists might be difficult in a chair or confined space. Although twists can be done without any particular arm position – just twist the head, neck, chest, abdomen and waist. The arm positions in these exercises and the previous one are additional: exercises for your arms.

Fingers on Shoulders (Base Position)

Bring your hands to your shoulders, touching your shoulders with your fingers and move your elbows back, bringing your shoulder blades closer together. Draw in your belly. Hold this position for a count of 10-30.

Base Position

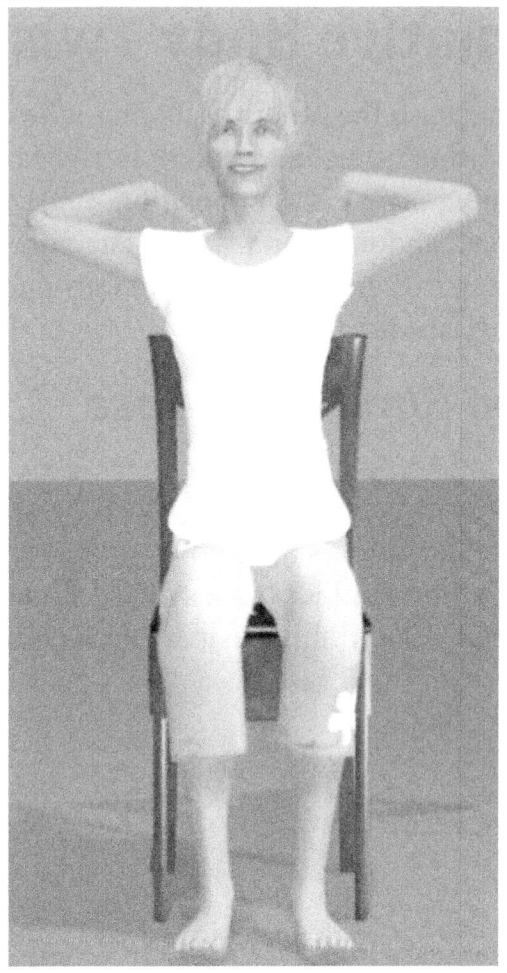

You may feel stretches in your shoulders and shoulder blades.

Twist Right

Still with your fingers on your shoulders twist your head, chest and abdomen to your right. Hold this position for a count of 10-30.

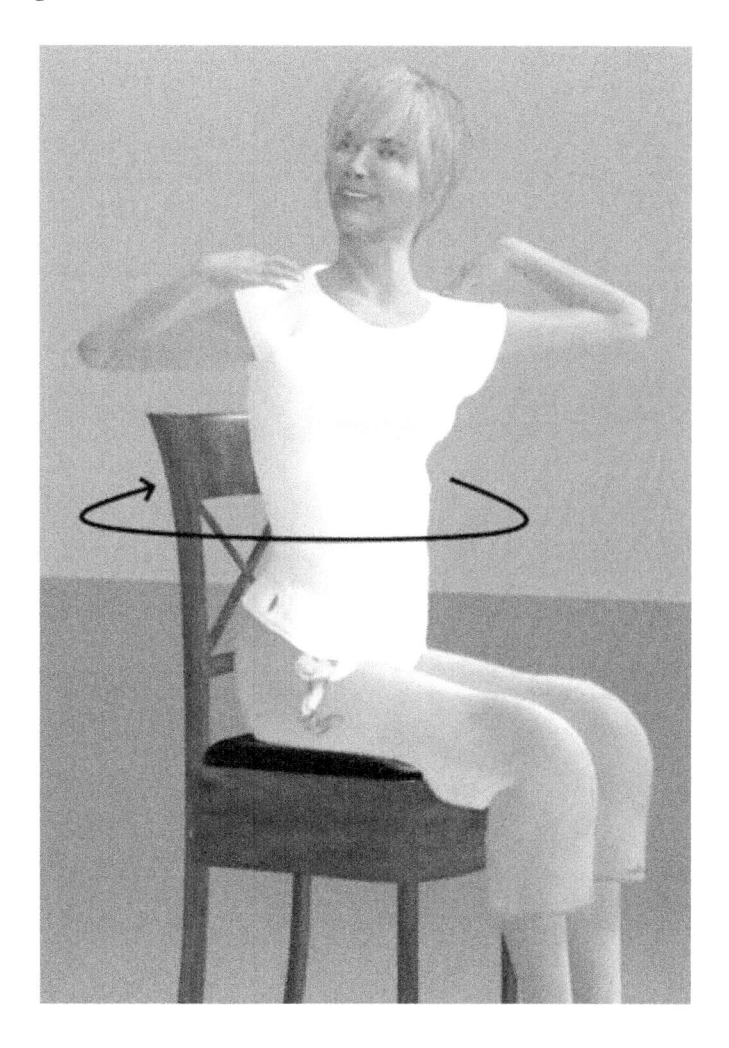

Twist Left

Turn your head, chest and abdomen to your left. Hold this position for a count of 10-30.

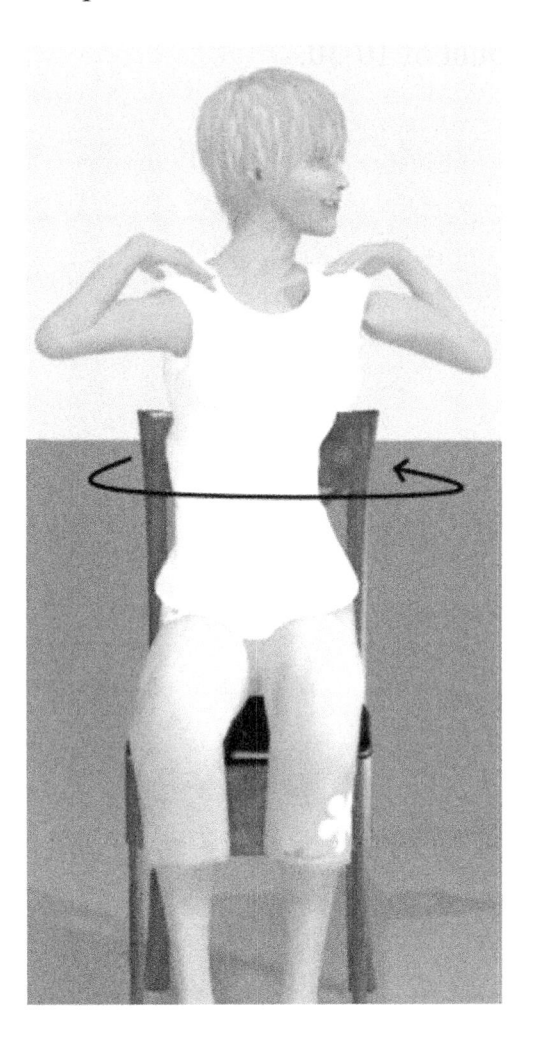

Did you pull your belly button in to stretch your abdominal muscles (abs)?

Belly Muscles (Abs)

Many of the exercises in this book work your belly muscles.

Breathe out so your belly is drawn in. You can put a hand on your belly to feel this happening.
Keep breathing in shorter breaths and keep your belly muscles taut for a count of 5 (or more with practice).

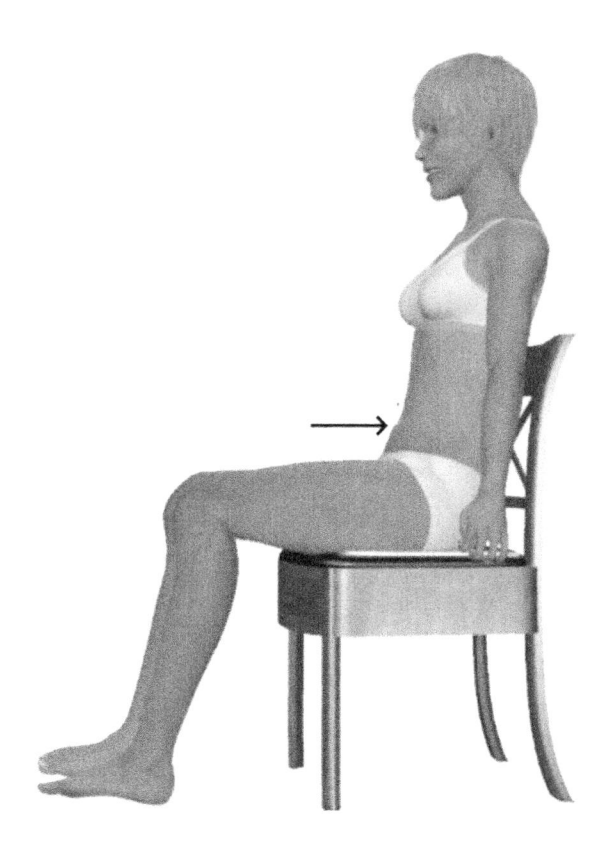

Then slowly release your muscles

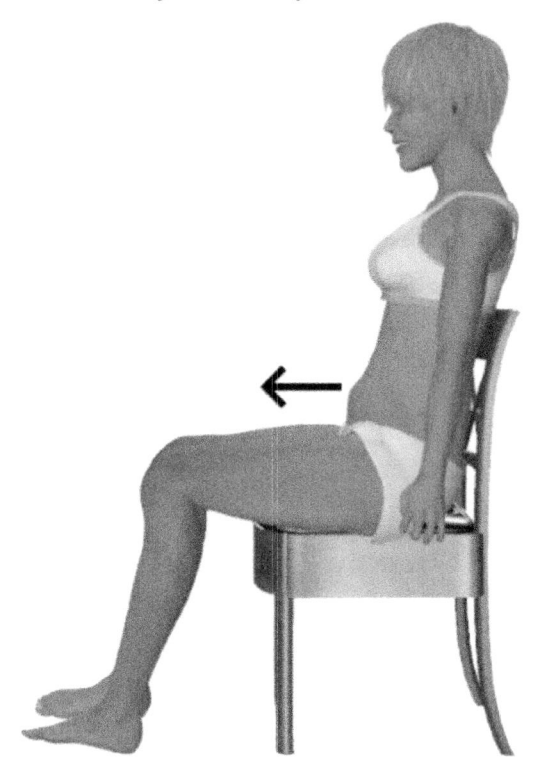

Repeat this belly in – hold for 5–and release, 5-20 or more times.

Another way to do this is to hold your belly stretched for a count of 10 to 30, remembering to breathe all the time. Repeat 5 times.

Arms and Shoulders

Hands Behind Head

Put your hands behind your head. Keep your spine and neck straight and move your elbows back as far as comfortable. Pull in your belly. Hold this pose for a count of 10-30.

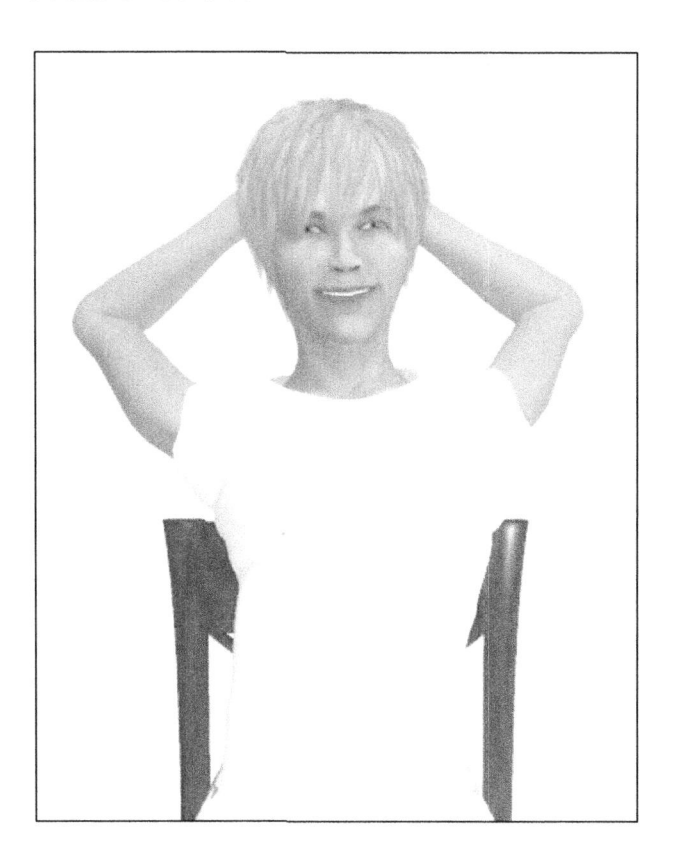

You should feel this pose in your shoulders mainly. The neck should feel comfortable. Of course, you also feel the stretch in your belly muscles.

Arms Up

Raise your arms above your head, keeping them straight, and touch your hands together, if possible. Hold the pose for a count of 10 to 30.

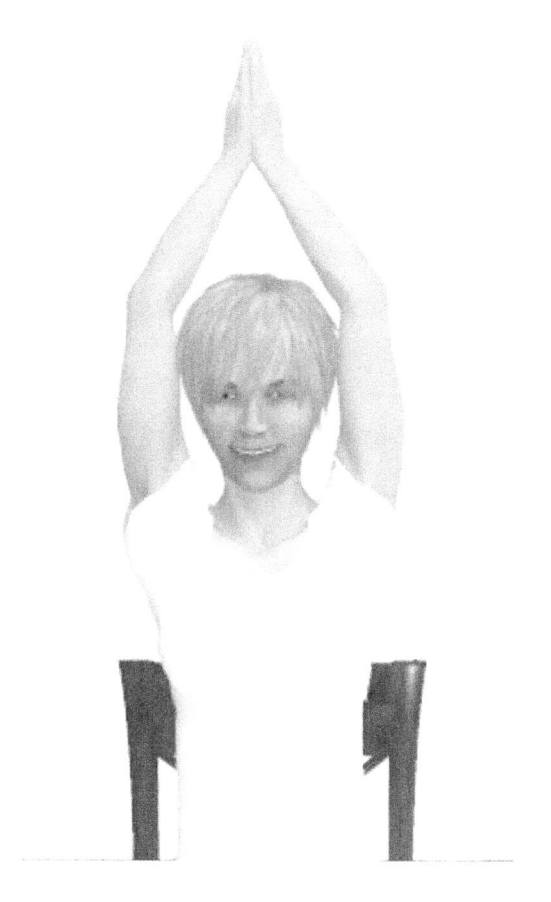

You may feel this pose mainly in the upper arms (biceps.)

Did you remember to keep your belly muscles stretched?

Arms T pose

Stretch out both arms to the side, making a T pose. (Or one arm at a time) and hold the pose for a count of 10-30.

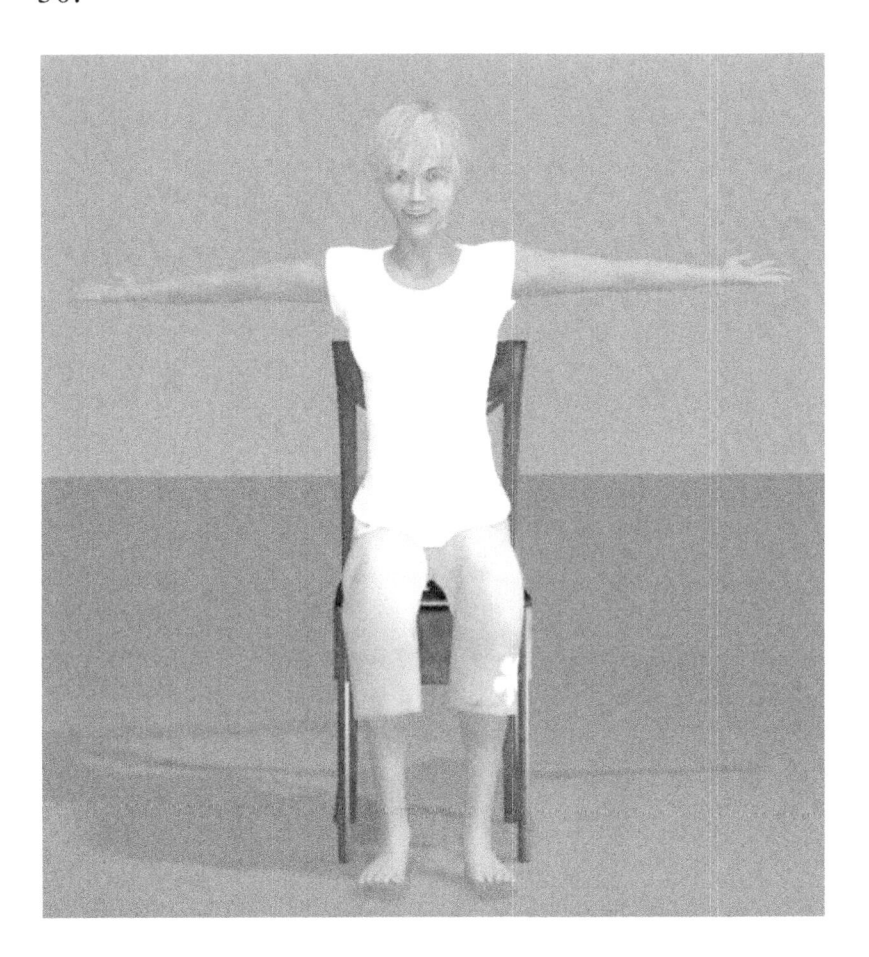

You may notice that your shoulders and arms are stretched by this pose.

Arms Straight Out

Stretch out both arms in front of you, keeping them as straight as you can, and letting your hands meet.

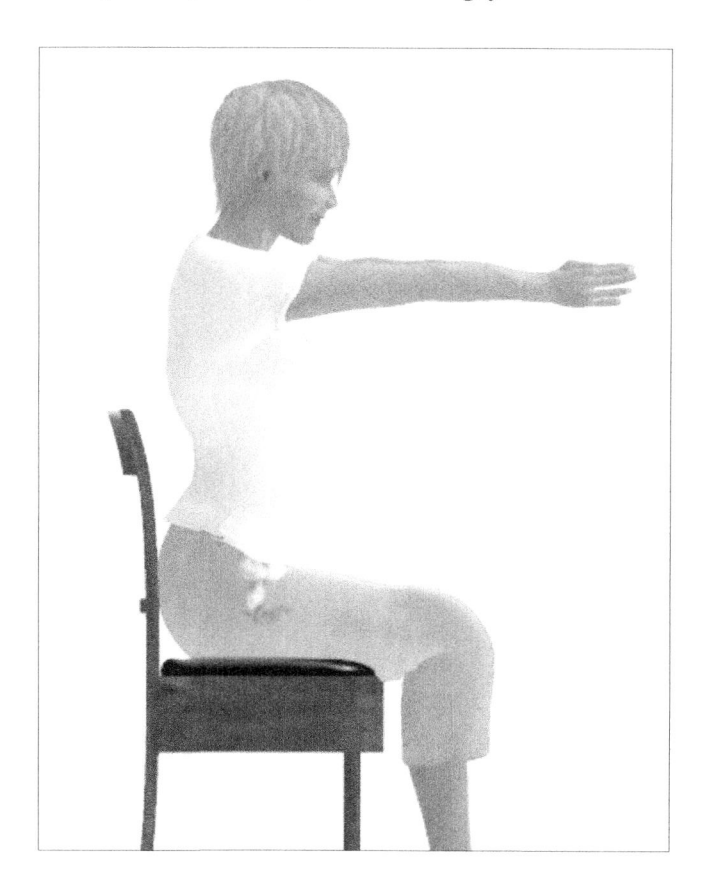

This pose may mainly affect your upper arms. Being mindful, ask yourself, "What other muscles are worked on by this pose?" scan your body to seek the answers.

Reversed Arms Stretch

Sit in the Base Position. Swing your arms back and up. Draw your shoulder blades together (or closer.) Your hands may meet or not at first. Do the best you can. Hold the position for a count of 10-30.

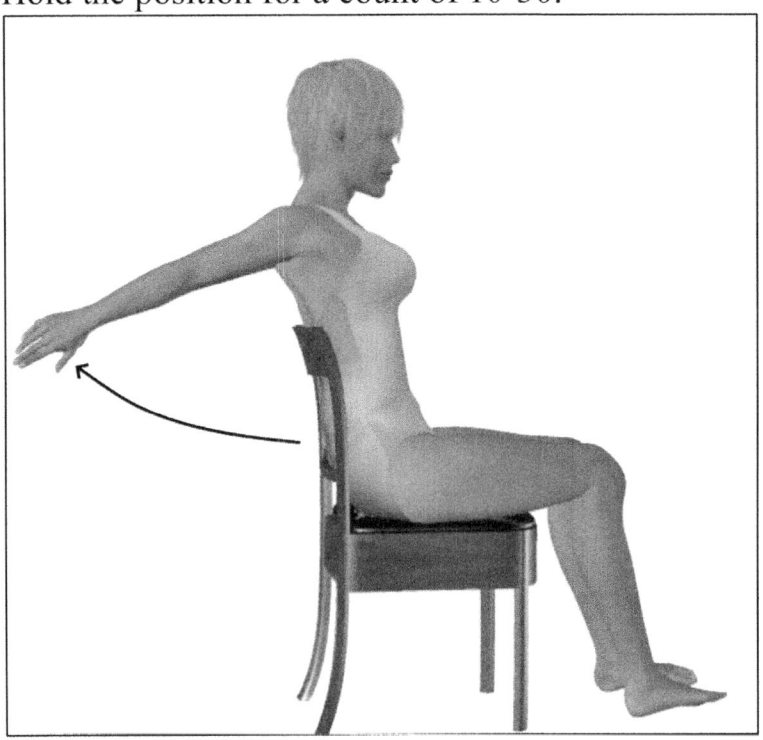

This pose works your shoulders, but it may also activate the muscles of your chest and your upper arms– and don't forget your belly. Ask yourself, "What other muscles are activated by this exercise?" Be aware of your body.

Shrugs

Raise your shoulders up towards your ears, as when shivering, or, well, shrugging.

Hold your raised shoulders for a count of 2-5, and repeat 10 times.

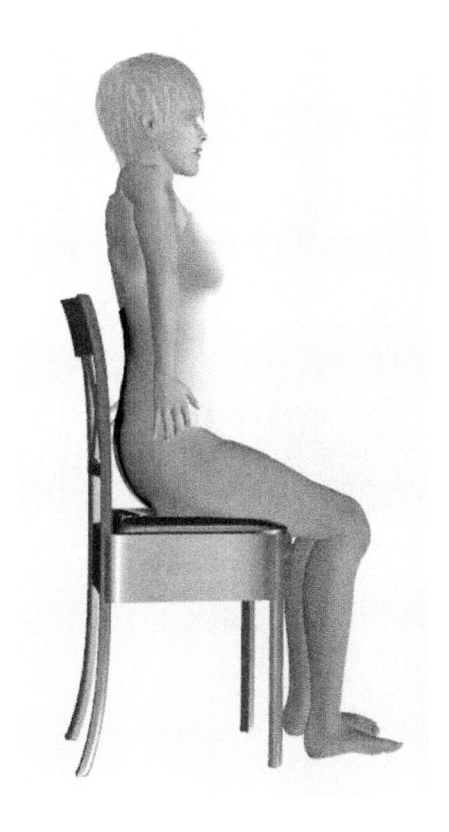

You may feel this in your upper back.

Elbow Circles

Stretch out your arms to your sides and bend your arms, putting your fingers on your shoulders. Circle each elbow for a count of 10-30. Repeat by circling in the opposite direction.

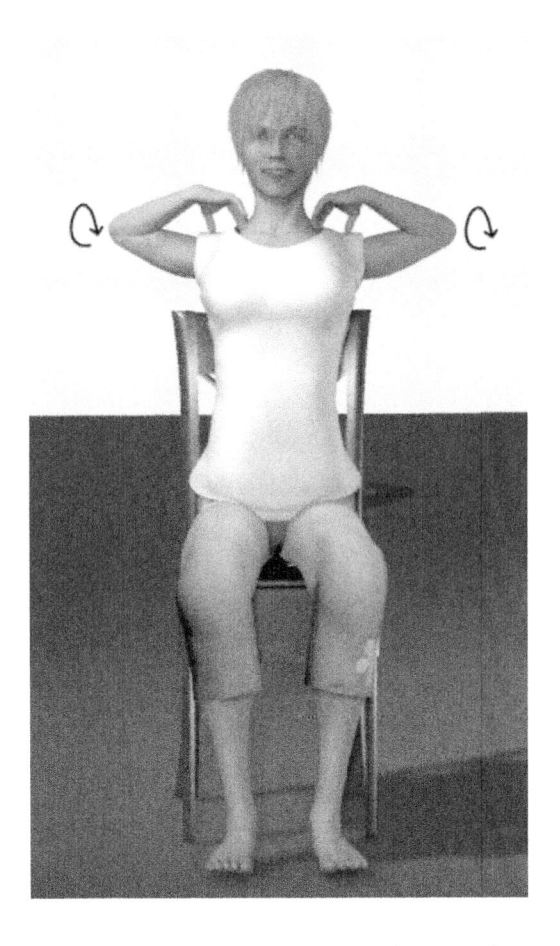

This is a different style of exercise – it uses movement, not holding a stretch.

Hands

As always do these slowly and comfortably, never with pain. Do not force any position against severe discomfort.

Hands Spread

Spread out your fingers, bending them back as is comfortable – don't forget your thumbs! Hold the stretch for a count of 10-30.

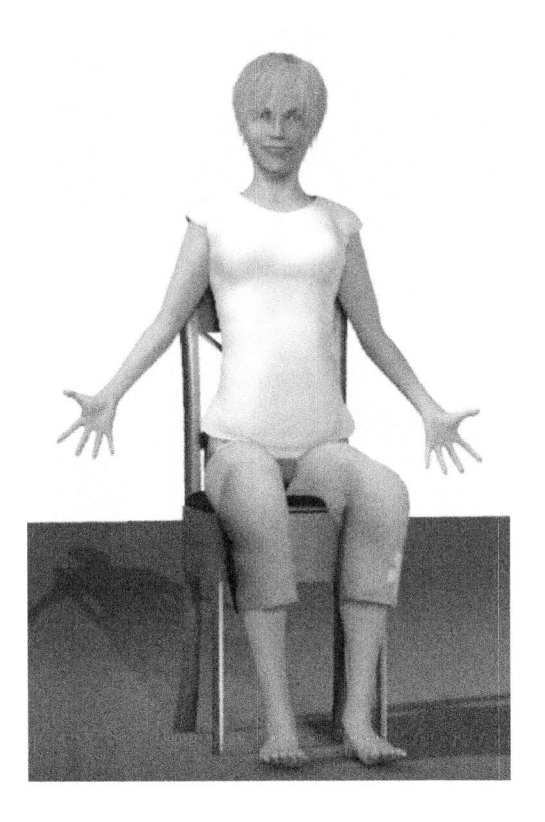

This and the next exercise are mainly concerned with your fingers, so the positions of the arms aren't important. However, as you get better at these hand exercises, you can incorporate them in other poses (as the yogis do.)

Hands Fists

Make your fists as tight as is comfortable and hold the pose for a count of 10-30.

You could alternate fists and spread, holding the pose for a count of 2-5, and repeating 10-30 times. These exercises can be done anytime.

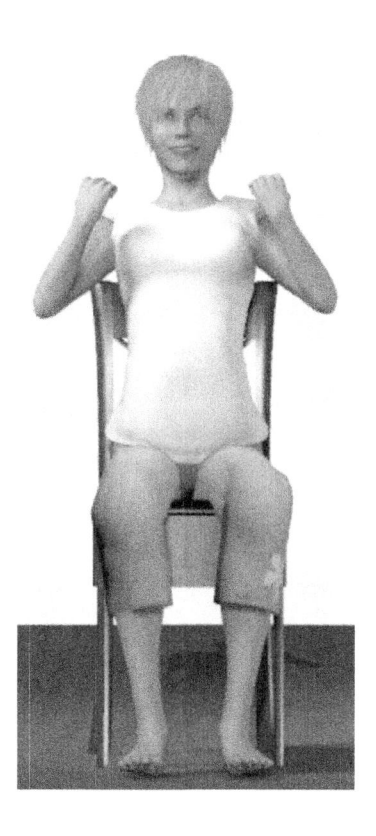

Prayer Hand Poses

You can hold each of these hand poses for a count of 10-30.

Prayer Hands Middle

Start from the middle position with your hands in a prayer pose. Gentle pressure to your fingers can be applied by any hand: your other hand resists.

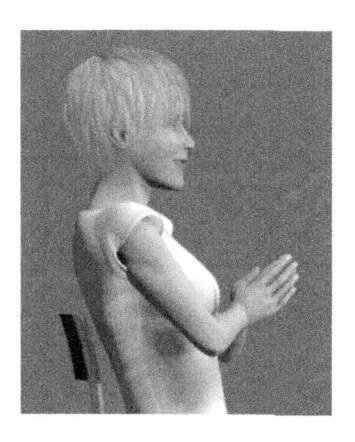

Prayer Hands Down

Bend the wrists down. Hold the pose for a count of 10-30.

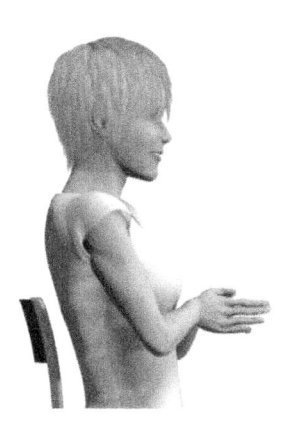

Prayer Hands Up

Bend your hands up. Hold the pose for a count of 10-30.

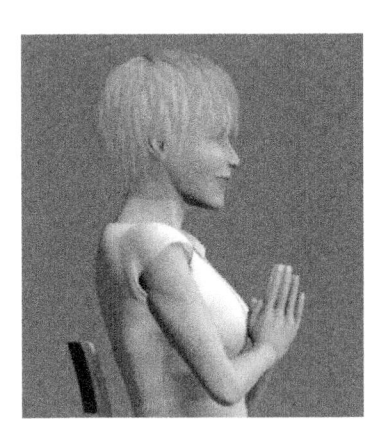

Prayer Hands Right

Bend your hands to your right. Gentle pressure to your fingers can be applied by your left hand. Hold the pose for a count of 10-30.

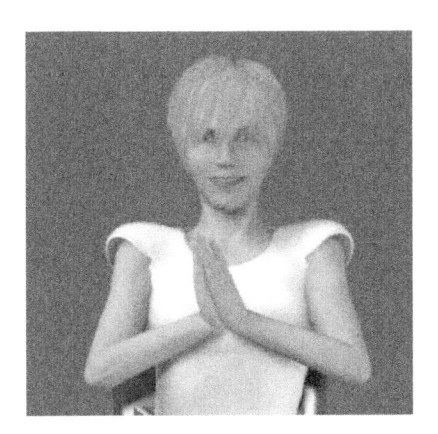

Prayer Hands Left

Bend your hands to your left. Hold the pose for a count of 10-30.

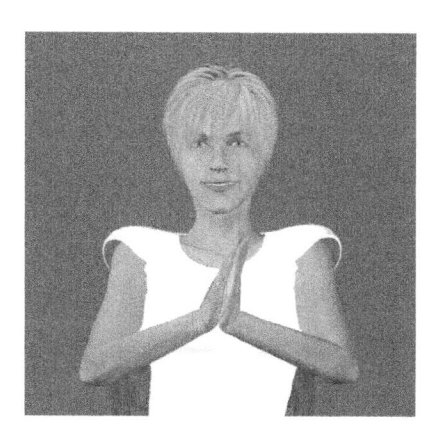

Neck

Finger-tip Pressure

If it is comfortable to do so, you can apply a *gentle*, *slow* finger-tip pressure with the appropriate hand. For example, in the Head Bent Back pose below. Hold these poses for a count of 10 to 30.

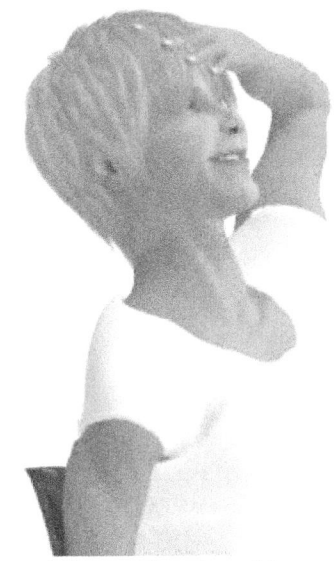

Head Bent Back with gentle finger-tip pressure.

Head Bent Back

Bend your neck back.

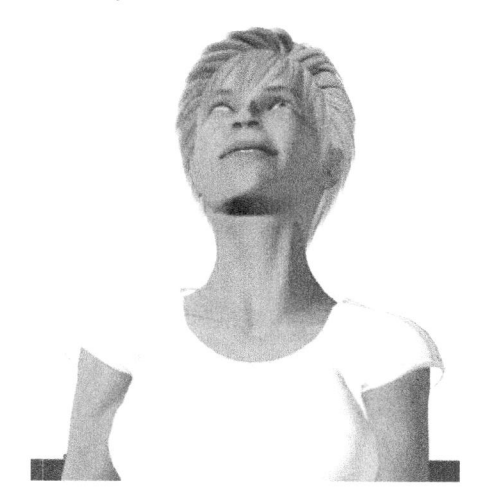

Head Bent Forward
Bend your neck forward.

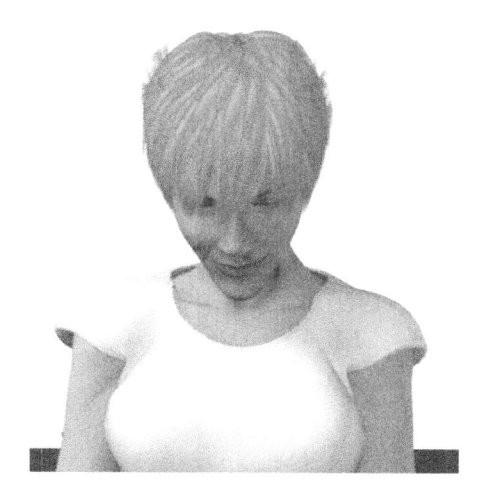

Look Left
Look as far to your left as is comfortable, turning your head slowly.

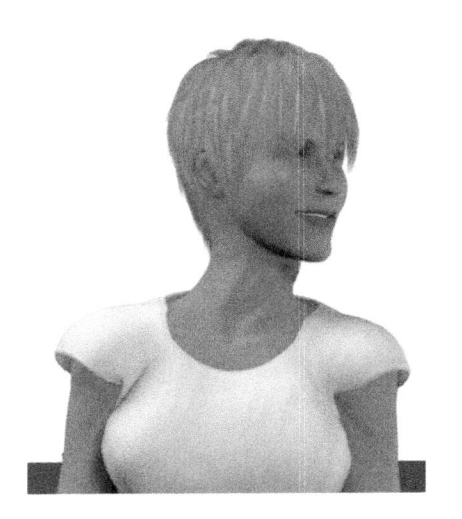

Look Right
Look as far to your right as is comfortable.

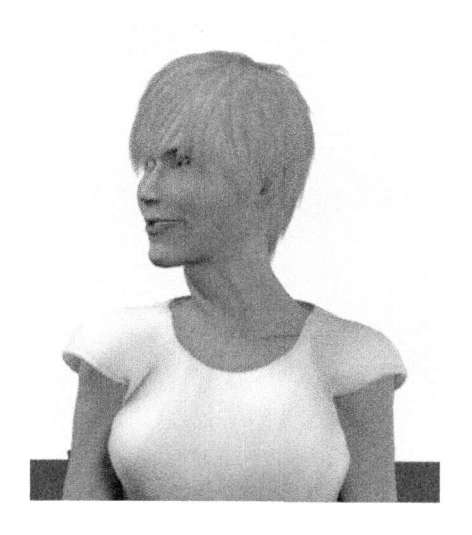

In the illustration below, the model is looking right applying gentle pressure with the finger tips of the left hand. If you wish, you can apply gentle pressure in all the above poses.

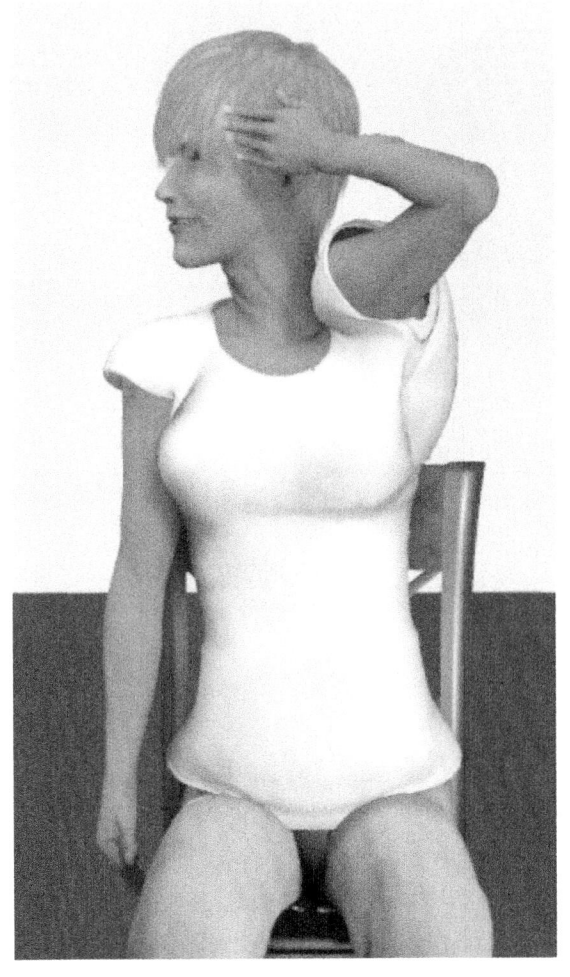

Eyes

Move your eyes smoothly in circles: first one way, then the other. For instance, clockwise and then anticlockwise. Repeat about 5 times.

Alternatively, you can stop at the extremes: Right, Up, Left and Bottom, holding the positions for a count of 10 or more.

Eyes Straight Ahead

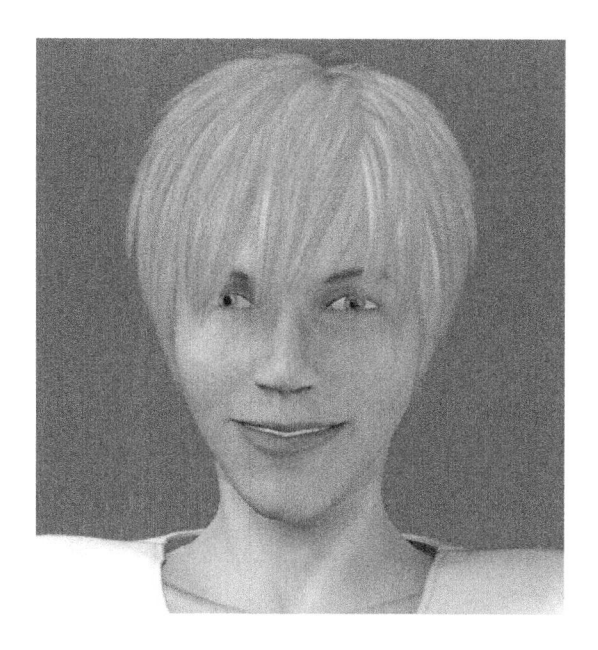

Eyes Right

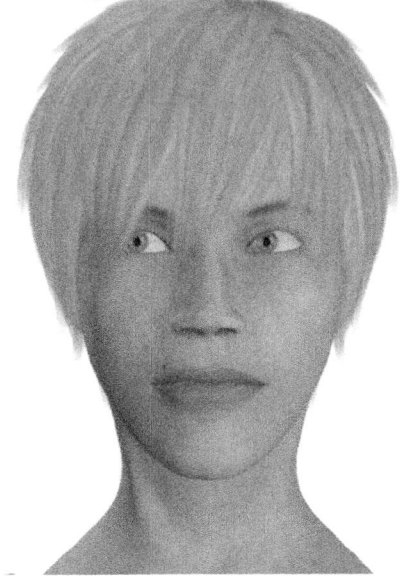

Eyes Up

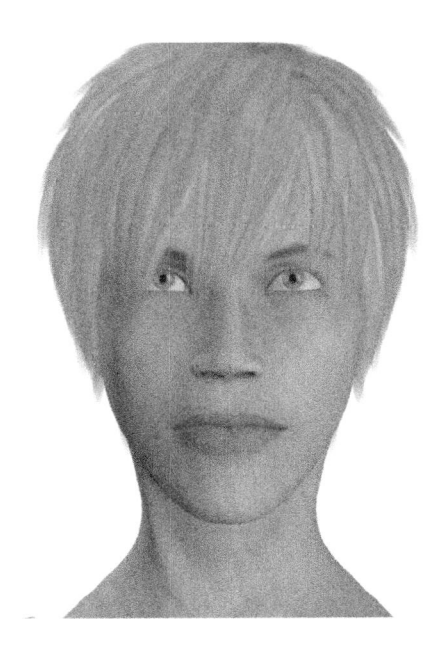

Eyes Left

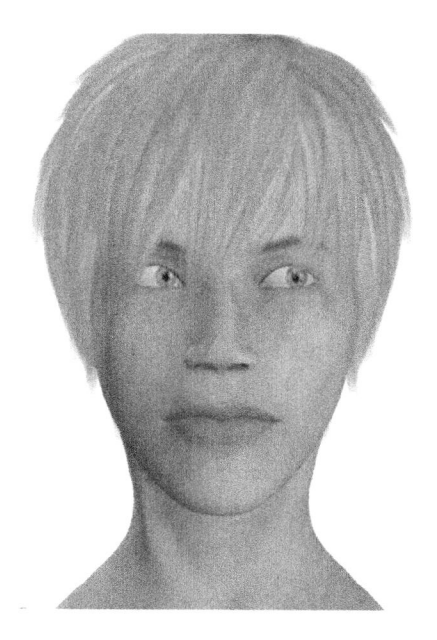

Eyes Down

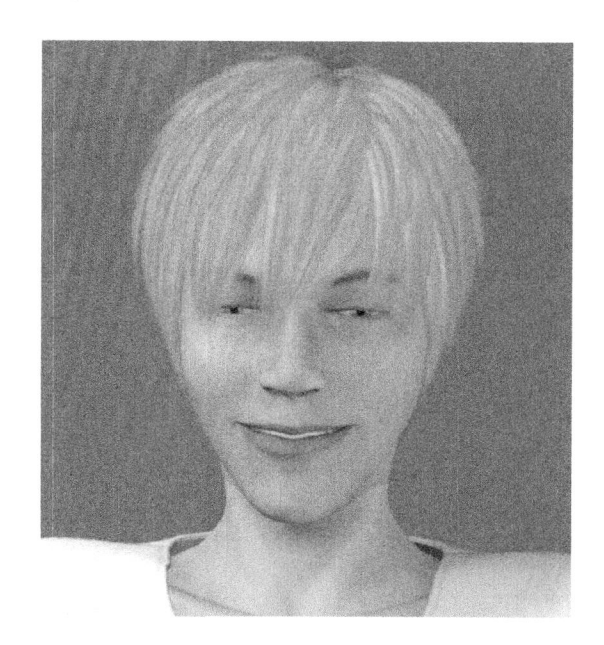

Heart and Lungs (Aerobic Exercises.)

These exercises stimulate your heart and lungs. Therefore, take advice from your health-care provider.

Raising Your Knees

This exercise is like *walking* or *jogging* in a chair. If you are unstable when standing or lack space, you can do this simply by raising one knee and then another, as in the Knee Up exercise.

Aerobic exercises stimulate the heart and lungs to work harder.

Health authorities recommend a half-hour walk for five days a week, or a jog for a similar period. This tells us that aerobic (heart and lung) exercises require a longer time than other exercises, but a beginner can start with what is comfortable and work up to longer periods. These, like the previous ones, can be thought of as strolling, marching or even jogging in a chair.

One way you can obtain aerobic effects is to raise one of your knees and then the other (without holding the extreme positions, as in the knees up exercises.)

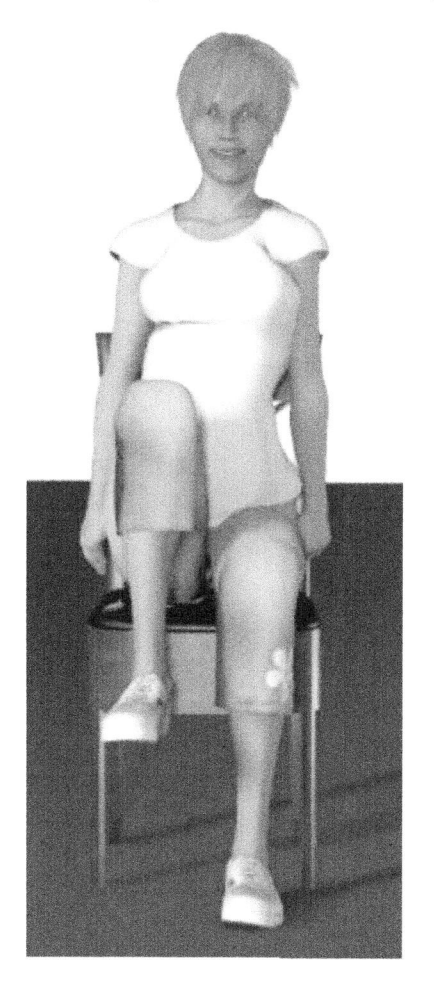

When learning these exercises, you should practise to discover what your manageable count is. (Count each knee raise, left or right as one.) This could be 30 to 100 or more. Or you could time yourself to find your best time, and use that (and a stopwatch.)

Also, you can do the exercises several times a day.

Raising Your Knees and Arms

If you need a stronger aerobic effect, then the previous exercise can be enhanced by raising your arms. You could also raise your arms above your head for a greater work out in the same time, but hasten slowly–avoid doing too much too soon.

Raise your right leg and arm:

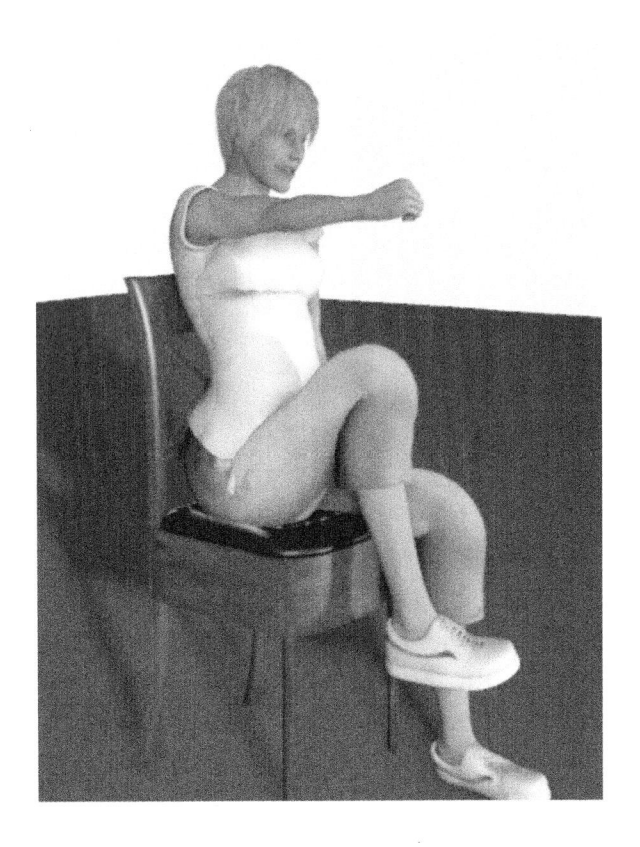

And then raise your left leg and arm.

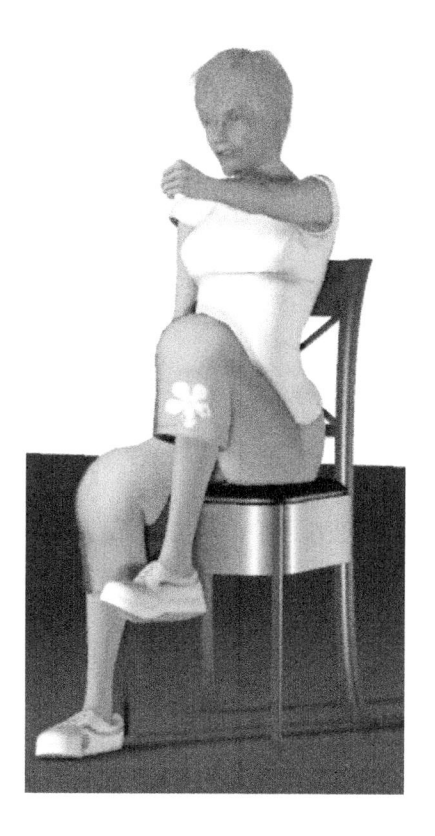

Work up from 30 to 50 knee raises (or fewer) as becomes comfortable.

The Future

I hope you have learned a bit about your body –even learning you have muscles you didn't know existed.

I hope you progress from these exercises, but they are useful in maintaining your everyday health.

Best wishes for health and happiness.

Printed in Great Britain
by Amazon